Boost Your Metabolism in 45 Minutes

Learn the Secret to Effective Weight Loss Fad Diets Won't Tell You About

By: Charles Williamson

9781681275062

PUBLISHERS NOTES

Disclaimer – Speedy Publishing LLC

This publication is intended to provide helpful and informative material. It is not intended to diagnose, treat, cure, or prevent any health problem or condition, nor is intended to replace the advice of a physician. No action should be taken solely on the contents of this book. Always consult your physician or qualified health-care professional on any matters regarding your health and before adopting any suggestions in this book or drawing inferences from it.

The author and publisher specifically disclaim all responsibility for any liability, loss or risk, personal or otherwise, which is incurred as a consequence, directly or indirectly, from the use or application of any contents of this book.

Any and all product names referenced within this book are the trademarks of their respective owners. None of these owners have sponsored, authorized, endorsed, or approved this book.

Always read all information provided by the manufacturers' product labels before using their products. The author and publisher are not responsible for claims made by manufacturers.

This book was originally printed before 2014. This is an adapted reprint by Speedy Publishing LLC with newly updated content designed to help readers with much more accurate and timely information and data.

Speedy Publishing LLC

40 E Main Street, Newark, Delaware, 19711

Contact Us: 1-888-248-4521

Website: http://www.speedypublishing.co

REPRINTED Paperback Edition: 9781681275062:

Manufactured in the United States of America

Dedication

This book is dedicated to Marina. You are an answered prayer. Thank you for coming into my life. .

Table of Contents

Chapter 1- Understanding the Metabolic Process 5

Chapter 2- How Your Metabolism Affects Weight Loss 11

Chapter 3- How to Boost Your Metabolism 15

Chapter 4- Exercise Smartly 19

Chapter 5- Your Lifestyle and Its Effects on Metabolism.............31

Chapter 6- Don't Eat Less, Just Eat Right...............................41

Chapter 7- Busting Myths about Diet.....................................51

About The Author...57

Chapter 1- Understanding the Metabolic Process

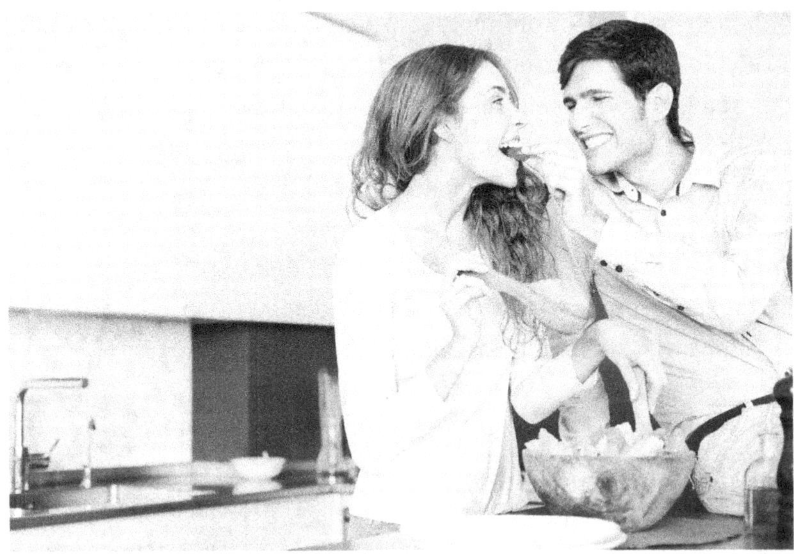

Some people think metabolism is a kind of organ, or a body part, that influences digestion.

Actually, the metabolism isn't a body part.

Metabolism is the process of transforming food (e.g. nutrients) into fuel (e.g. energy). The body uses this energy to conduct a vast array of essential functions.

In fact, your ability to read this page is driven by your metabolism.

If you had no metabolism you wouldn't be able to move.

In fact, long before you realized that you couldn't move a finger or lift your foot, your internal processes would have stopped, because the basic building blocks of life – circulating blood, transforming oxygen into carbon dioxide, expelling potentially lethal wastes through the kidneys and so on – all of these depend on metabolism.

Although we think of our metabolism as a single function, it's really a catch-all term for countless functions that are taking place inside the body. Every second of every minute of every day of your life numerous chemical conversions are taking place through metabolism, or metabolic functioning.

In a certain light, the metabolism has been referred to as a harmonizing process that manages to achieve two critical bodily functions that seem to be at odds with each other.

How It Works

First, let us start with the act of eating. As you chew and swallow your food, it goes down to your digestive tract. Digestive enzymes then break down your food – carbohydrates to glucose, fats into fatty acids, and protein into amino acids. After the nutrients are effectively broken down, they are absorbed by the bloodstream and are carried over to the cells. Other enzymes plus hormones then work to either convert these nutrients into cells or building blocks for tissues or release them as an energy supply for the body's immediate use.

The Types and Components of Metabolism

There are two basic metabolic processes – one is constructive, and is responsible for building and storing energy for the body. The other is destructive, though in a positive sense, as it breaks down nutrient molecules to release energy.

The constructive metabolic process is called anabolism, while the destructive process is called catabolism.

Charles Williamson
Anabolism vs. Catabolism

Our bodies are continually creating more cells to replace dead or dysfunctional cells. For example, if you cut your finger, your body starts the process of creating skin cells to clot the blood and start the healing process instantly. This creation process is a metabolic response, and is called anabolism.

On the other hand, there is the exact opposite activity taking place in other parts of the body. Instead of building cells and tissue the body is breaking down energy so the body can function.

For example, as you exercise, your body temperature rises and your heart beat increases. As this happens, your body requires more oxygen, so your breathing increases. If your body couldn't adjust to this enhanced requirement for oxygen, you would collapse. And all of this requires additional energy.

Presuming that you aren't overdoing it, your body will begin converting food into energy in a metabolic process called catabolism.

Your metabolism is a constant process that works in two seemingly opposite ways: anabolism uses energy to create cells, and catabolism breaks down cells to create energy.

There are three further components to catabolism and these are:

1. Basal metabolism

Sometimes called resting metabolism, this is the metabolism component responsible for keeping you alive by ensuring normal body functions. Even if you were bedridden the whole day, basal metabolism is still at work.

Basal metabolism is metabolism's main component, as 60 to 70 percent of the calories from the food you eat are used for this. People who want to lose weight usually aim for a higher basal metabolic rate (BMR).

2. Physical movement

This can range from a simple moving of your fingers to strenuous exercise. Usually 25 percent of the calories you consume go here.

3. Thermic effect of food

This indicates the digestion and processing of the food you take in. Normally, ten percent of the calories of the food you eat are burned through this.

Thus, taking all this into account, here is our metabolism formula:

Calories from Food = Calories Expended From Basal Metabolism (60-70%) + Calories Expended By Physical Movement (25%) + Calories Expended Digesting Food (10%)

What Affects Your Metabolism?

Your metabolic rate, or how fast or slow your metabolism works, is influenced by a number of factors:

1.Genetics

Yes, metabolic rate is also inherited. Sometimes this makes an entire world of difference between a person who can eat almost everything and not gain an ounce and a person who easily balloons after indulging just once.

2.Age

The younger you are, the faster your metabolism is. Metabolism slows down as you age. Women's metabolic rate starts falling at the age of 30; for men, decline starts later at the age of 40.

3.Gender

Men have a faster metabolic rate – usually 10-15 percent faster – than women because their bodies have a larger muscle mass. Muscle plays a key role in fast metabolism.

4.Amount of lean body mass

As already mentioned above, more muscle = faster metabolism.

5.Diet

Some foods will help you, some will only harm you. While timing is not everything, when you eat also greatly affects your metabolism.

6.Stress level

Stress is inversely proportional to metabolism. The more stress you are subjected to, the lower your metabolism.

7.Hormones

Specific hormones metabolize specific nutrients. How well the hormones work, then, directly affects metabolism. To a certain extent, diet and stress levels affect the hormones involved in metabolism, as you will find out later. Hormonal disorders or imbalances can affect metabolism as well.

Looking at all these factors that influence metabolism, you now probably have a general idea of what you need to do to increase your metabolism – accept the things you cannot change, and work on those that you can!

Chapter 2- How Your Metabolism Affects Weight Loss

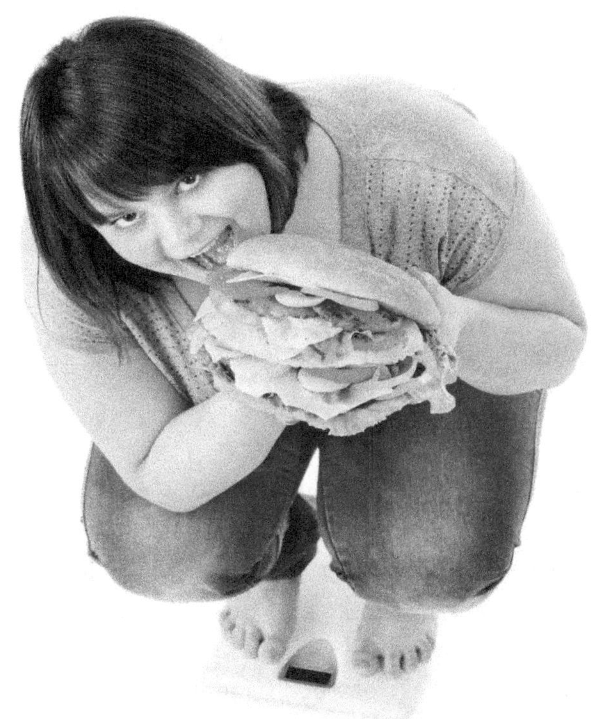

Calories

Calories are simply units of measure, not actual things. They are labels like an inch which really isn't anything, but it measures the distance between two points.

So what do calories measure? Energy.

Your body creates energy from the food you eat, whether it's healthy food or not. It creates energy from fruits and vegetables using the same process that it uses to create energy from chocolate bars and candy.

Boost Your Metabolism in 45 Minutes

While you know it's better for your body to get energy from fruit and vegetables, your body doesn't evaluate the food. It creates energy from whatever you feed it.

It sounds strange, but the body really doesn't care. To the body, energy is energy. It takes whatever it gets, and doesn't really know that some foods are healthier than others. It's kind of like a garbage disposal: it takes what you put down it, whether it should go down or not.

So let's apply this to the body, and to weight gain. When the body receives a calorie it must do something with that energy. If a carrot delivers 100 calories to the body, it has to accept those 100 calories. The same goes for 200 calories from chocolate bars and candy.

The body does one of two things to the energy, it either metabolizes it via anabolism, or it metabolizes it via catabolism. That is, it will either convert the energy (calories) into cells/tissue, or it will use that energy (calories) to break down cells.

When there is an excess of energy, and the body can't use this energy to deal with any needs at the time, it will be forced to create cells with that extra energy. It has to.

It doesn't necessarily want to, but after figuring out that the energy can't be used to do anything (such as help you exercise or digest some food), it has to turn it into cells through anabolism.

And those extra cells? Yup, you guessed it: added weight.

In a nutshell, the whole calorie/metabolism/weight gain thing is really just about excess energy. When there are too many calories in the body, they are transformed into fat.

Sometimes those extra calories are transformed into muscle. In fact, muscles require calories to maintain their mass, so people with strong muscle tone burn calories without actually doing anything; their metabolism burns it for them.

This is the primary reason why exercising and building lean muscle is part of an overall program to boost your metabolism. The more lean muscle you have, the more places excess calories can go before they're turned into fat.

Fat Cells Are Not Permanent

There's a nasty rumor floating around that fat cells are permanent. Unfortunately, the rumor is true. Most experts agree that once fat cells have been created, they're permanent. But this doesn't spell doom and gloom for those of us who could stand to drop a few pounds. Even though experts believe that fat cells are permanent, they also agree that fat cells can be shrunk. So even if the number of fat cells in your body remains the same, their size, appearance and percentage of your overall weight, can be reduced.

But it's Not All about Weight Loss

It's not all about weight loss, though discussions on metabolism seem to focus almost exclusively on this concept. In fact, even if you feel that your weight is perfectly fine, you have a lot to gain by increasing your metabolism. Following a list of the benefits you stand to gain by applying the advice in this book:

1. Lose weight. Let's start with the most obvious benefit. By increasing your metabolism, particularly your BMR, you will burn more calories just by doing the activities you usually do. Even while you lie in bed and stare at the ceiling or even while you are sleeping, your body is working to burn the calories you consume.

With an increase in metabolism, you can actually shed one or two pounds a week. Best of all, the results are long-term, unlike a quick-fix diet! Now, isn't that more satisfying – and easier – than going on a fad diet?

2. Eat more without worrying about it. Since you burn calories faster now, you can eat more without feeling guilty. This does not mean overindulging or snacking on junk food, though. But in general, you can be less concerned about the quantity of food you eat.

3. Feel more energized. People with faster metabolism report having more energy. With a faster metabolism, your body is performing efficiently to release the energy you need to get going.

4. Look better. The skin of people with a fast metabolism is brighter and more radiant. Their faces are pinkish, more alive with color. With a faster metabolism, you will not only feel good but also look good!

5. Be healthier overall. Your body functions more efficiently with a faster metabolism. Digestion, absorption of nutrients and blood circulation are improved. And your body won't need as much sleep as you did before to feel refreshed the next day.

In sum, expect a faster metabolism to make you look and feel more wonderful.

Chapter 3- How to Boost Your Metabolism

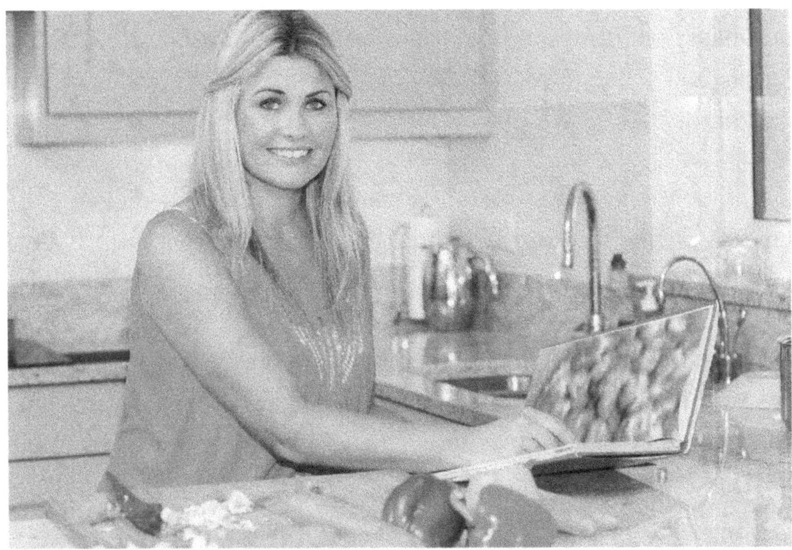

Chances are you've tried to boost your metabolism at least once in your life. Perhaps you weren't quite certain what a metabolism was, or didn't know how to accomplish your goals.

Maybe you started a rigorous exercise program of jogging and muscle toning. Or you started eating several small portions a day, rather than three large traditional meal-sized portions. Maybe you started taking all kinds of supplements that promised to boost your metabolism.

The thing is all of these methods can work.

Exercise, eating strategically, and ensuring that your body has catabolism-friendly supplements are three of many generally good weight loss ideas.

So what's the problem?

The problem is, many of us have no real scientific understanding of what, how, or why these methods boost metabolism.

For example, a person may start a vigorous exercise program that includes significant aerobic cardiovascular movement, such as jogging or cycling. After a week, that person may notice a drop in weight.

But is this due to a boosted metabolism? Maybe - maybe not. Could it be due to water loss through perspiration that hasn't been adequately replenished? Maybe - maybe not.

Many people risk their health, because they don't quite understand the tips, strategies, and techniques of boosting their metabolism. There are eleven key ideas to do this. And these are broken them down into 3 broad categories for easier reference:

1. Exercise

2. Lifestyle

3. Diet

As you go through each of the 11 key points, you'll certainly note that there is some overlap between them. For example, it's hard to imagine that introducing exercise into your life isn't a lifestyle choice.

Don't get bogged down in the categories; they are merely provided to help organize these points, and to help you easily refer to them in the future. The important thing is to understand each of the 14 points, and evaluate how you can responsibly integrate them into your life.

You are probably wondering what all this has to do with mindset. Why not go directly to the advice for increasing your metabolism?

The reason is that you need to be prepared for what lies ahead. Boosting your metabolism is a serious business. It is not like a quick-fix diet where you need only exert effort for a few weeks – and for some diets, even for a few days.

Boosting your metabolism is about changing your lifestyle and habits. Though you may choose to start with small changes, you will still be changing the way of life you have become used to – and it may feel uncomfortable at first. Boosting your metabolism requires discipline and consistency in your actions. And since you are expecting long-term results, you are likewise expected to make a long-term investment.

From here on, please look at the advice I will be presenting as an entire package or program. You cannot do only some of them and still get the same results. The tips here follow the gestalt principle – the whole is greater than the sum of the parts. Trust that the components of the program all work harmoniously to deliver your desired result.

So now I want you to close your eyes and imagine yourself – really imagine! What you will be like after this program has started to take effect on you. How will you look? How will you feel?

Then, do the same process for your expectations after three months, then six months – or even a year, if you can. Note the differences you see and feel.

It's a good idea to write down your expected outcome. This will help you get through the program, especially when you are having a difficult time sticking to the changes you previously committed to.

Congratulations! You have just begun with the end in your mind. This will greatly help you along the way to your goal of firing up your metabolism.

Chapter 4- Exercise Smartly

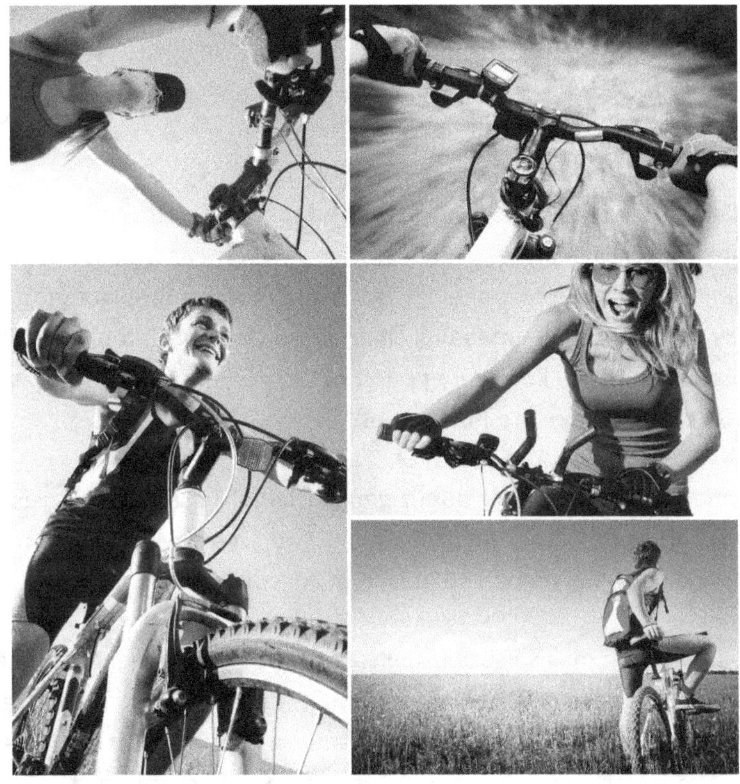

Notice that I mentioned smart, not hard. Though some exercises here may be high-intensity and may indeed be hard for you, you need not work as long and as hard as you may think. The goal here is to fire up your metabolism with an exercise program that takes the shortest time and the least effort possible without sacrificing results.

The two elements in this exercise program are strength and resistance training for building lean muscle mass and interval training for speeding up the metabolic process in general.

Strength and Resistance Training

The exercises under this training program are designed to literally build strength and resistance, as the name suggests. Tension is applied on the muscles to achieve this. The end result is increased muscle mass in your body.

Building muscle is important as more muscle in your body means more calories burned. Fitness trainer and consultant Robert Reames gives a perfect analogy by calling muscles fireplaces in the body that burn fuel – meaning calories. So the more fireplaces, the more fuel burned. For every pound of muscle added to your body, 40-50 calories more are burned per day.

Women need not worry about gaining large, unsightly muscles – your bodies are different from men. Your muscles will only add definition to your shape and in fact, make you look sexier.

While building muscles are usually associated with weight training, this is not always the case. There are in fact several exercises that do not require weights at all. If you are on a tight budget, you can in fact do exercises with no weights at all. For best results, though, do a combination of strength exercises with equipment and without equipment.

For clear differentiation, let us discuss weight lifting exercises first.

Weight lifting is a convenient muscle-building exercise as it applies tension to your muscles through an external source, the weights. You can also easily measure your progress as the number of pounds or grams is indicated on each weight. As your body adjusts and strengthens, you can add more weights or replace your current weights with heavier ones. To determine how many grams or pounds your weights should have, try them out first. The best weights for you are those that put tension in your muscles but do not make you feel fatigued.

The best exercises for achieving faster results for boosting metabolism are those that work several muscles in your body together. It's not a problem if you want to focus on a particular muscle, though, for example, if you want to tone or sculpt a specific body part.

There are many weight-lifting exercises you can choose from to include in your routine, but here are some basic examples:

1. Bench press – This is a multi-joint exercise, working the major muscles of the shoulders, chest and triceps. To do this, lie on a bench and hold the weight over your chest with your elbows bent at 90 degrees. "Press" the weight up until your arms straighten, then lower it slowly back to your starting position.

2. Chest fly – This works the chest, with an emphasis on outer muscles. Lie on a bench with your weights held overhead, palms facing inward. Lower the weights to your sides up to shoulder level, with your elbows slightly bent. Slowly bring the weights up, back to starting position.

3. Bicep curl – This is one of the most basic weight lifting exercises. This puts effort on the biceps, as the name suggests. To do this, hold the weights with your palms facing out. Bend your elbows to bring the weights to your shoulders without touching them. Slowly lower the weights down, but do not straighten the arm out totally to keep a level of tension.

4. Concentration curl – This also works the biceps. Kneel on one leg using the leg opposite the hand you are working with. Hold one weight with your working hand and put the other hand on your

waist. Place the back of the upper arm of your working hand on the inner thigh of the other leg. You can lean into that leg to raise your elbow a little. Raise the weight to the front of your shoulder and then slowly lower the arm until almost straight.

5. Overhead press – This works the shoulder muscles. Stand or sit straight and hold your weights with your elbows bent and your hands in front of your eyes. Bring the weights over your head while keeping your back straight. Slowly bring the weights down to starting position.

Strength exercises without weights can be combined with weight lifting exercises for your routine.

Here are some examples:

1.Squat

A squat is a multi-joint exercise working the hamstrings, quadriceps, gluteals, and the lower back. In fact, this is one of the most effective strength exercises without weights. From a standing position, slowly lower your body until your knees bend at a 90-degree angle. Keep your feet flat on the floor while doing this. Return to a standing position slowly as well.

2.Pushup

This is also a very typical but effective strength and resistance exercise. While the basic one works well, adding complexity can work more muscles.

For example, you can do pushups between two chairs. These work the chest and the triceps. Place both feet on a stable chair and then place both hands on separate chairs. The two chairs your hands are resting on can have a gap of 60 centimeters. The chair with your feet should align with the middle of the other two chairs. Your body should be stretched naturally from the chair at your feet to the chairs in front. Slowly bring your chest down – beyond the surface of the chairs if you can!

3.Crunch

Yes, the basic crunch is a strength exercise, although it works mostly for the abs only. But though the crunch is well-known, not everyone knows how to do it properly. To do this correctly, lie on the floor or a mat with your knees bent and your feet flat on the floor. You may put your hands behind your head. Raise your upper body – but lead with your chest – upwards until you feel your abs contract. To keep the tension, do not raise your body up to 90 degrees. Again, to keep tension, when you bring your body down, do not let it rest on the floor. Instead, keep yourself a bit elevated from the floor.

For variety in exercises and for working different sets of muscles, you can also try working out with different equipment like exercise balls. In planning your routine for strength exercises, refer to the body's muscle groups below and determine which you want to work on. Remember, though, that multi-joint exercises are still best to achieve faster metabolism.

1. Biceps – These are found at the front of your upper arm.

2. Triceps – These are at the back of your upper arm.

3. Deltoids – These are the caps of your shoulders.

4. The Pectoralis major – This is the large, fan-shaped muscle on the front of your upper chest.

5. Rhomboids – These are muscles in the middle of your upper back and located between the shoulder blades.

6. Trapezius – This is on your upper back, sometimes called 'traps'. The upper trapezius, in particular, runs from the back of your neck to your shoulder.

7. Latisimus dorsi – These are large muscles that go down the middle of your back. When exercised well, they give your back an attractive V shape, giving the illusion of a smaller waist.

8. Lower back – This comprises the erector spine muscles that enable back extension. This also helps in maintaining good posture.

9. Abdominals – Of course! This is where the belly fat usually goes, the flab you want to banish forever. The abdominals are composed of the external oblique, which trace paths down the sides and the front of the abdomen, and the rectus abdominus, a flat muscle running across the abdomen.

10. Gluteals – Also called "glutes," the main muscle here is the gluteus maximus, the muscle on your buttocks.

11. Quadriceps – These muscles go up the front of your thigh.

12. Hamstrings – These are on the back of your thighs.

13. Hip abductors and adductors – These are located at your inner and outer thigh. Abductors are on the outside, moving the leg away from your body. On the other hand, adductors are on the inside, pulling the leg to the center of your body.

14. Calf – The calf muscles are on the back of the lower leg. The two calf muscles are the gastrocnemius and the soleus. The former

gives the calf a stable, round shape while the soleus is a flat muscle below the gastrocnemius.

After choosing your exercises, you must think about the level of intensity and the duration of your exercises. The number of repetitions and sets actually depends on your level of tolerance – fatigue is a sign that you have overtaxed yourself. Let yourself feel the "burn" in your muscles or the soreness but do not push yourself more than you can go. In general, though, the American College of Sports Medicine recommends three sets or more of strength exercises with six to eight repetitions for each set for building muscle. If you are a beginner, though, it may take time before you reach this level. Not more than a 45-second rest should be taken between sets for best results in increasing metabolism.

Your exercise routine can last for only 30 minutes or less and still achieve optimum results.

At this point, I want to emphasize that strength and resistance exercises are the best and healthiest way to build muscles. Do not ever look for shortcuts, like performance-enhancing drugs or steroids with growth hormones. While they may help increase your muscle mass, they can have side effects such as heart attacks, liver damage, and even premature death. It is best for you to stick to the healthy and proven methods in building muscles.

The benefits of strength exercises are also numerous and not merely confined to boosting metabolism. They lower blood pressure, improve balance and flexibility, increase your stamina for other activities, and reduce your risk of injury – as these are strength exercises, they in fact strengthen your muscles and bones!

Interval Training

Yes, these exercises are about "intervals," particularly the intervals of high-intensity exercise and rest. In this training, you do a cardiovascular exercise at the highest intensity you can manage, then shift to a moderate intensity, do high intensity again, and then moderate, and so on. Reames calls this "metabolic burst" training, as the sudden burst you do in the high-intensity exercise also results in a burst of calorie-burning. Because of the sudden "burst" you give to your body, it also suddenly releases energy. The rest period, meanwhile, is essential for the body to get rid of the waste products in the muscles you are using in the exercise. It is important to keep a moderate intensity of exercise and not go into total rest. This is to ensure that the release of energy is continuous.

Interval training can be done for almost any type of cardiovascular exercise – running, biking, swimming, and more. For running, the rest period can be brisk walking; for biking and swimming, the activity can be done at a slower but moderate pace. The high-intensity and moderate-intensity exercise can also be slightly different. For example, the high-intensity exercise may be briskly walking up the stairs while the low-intensity exercise may be brisk walking on a flat surface.

Each interval should last between one to four minutes. The rest period can be shorter or longer than your high-intensity exercise, depending on your condition. Doing your interval training routine for a total of 30 minutes already achieves optimal results. Just ensure that your moderate-intensity exercise really still has intensity while allowing your body to rest for the next burst of high-intensity exercise. Perform your personal best for the high-intensity exercise – being almost out of breath is a good sign.

A more accurate way of determining the highest level of intensity you can manage is by calculating your maximum heart rate. To get your maximum heart rate, simply subtract your age from 220. During exercise, a heart rate monitor will come in handy although this is optional. To monitor your heart rate manually, find your pulse in your wrist then count the number of beats within six seconds. Put the number zero at the end of that. If you counted 16 beats, your pulse rate is 160 beats per minute. Your pulse rate after high-intensity exercise should be 75-85 percent of your maximum heart rate. Your pulse rate during moderate-intensity exercise should always be greater than your resting heart rate or your normal heart rate when you are not doing any exercise. Again, to get your resting heart rate, get your pulse rate while you are not doing exercise.

For those who want to boost metabolism primarily to lose weight, here's the good news: after a few weeks of interval training, expect even your normal exercise with moderate intensity to burn more fat than usual. A study by exercise scientist Jason Talanian supports this claim. After seven interval workouts distributed over two weeks, subjects increased their fat burning by 36 percent through normal cycling exercises only.

Also, according to Reames, after interval training comes the "metabolic after burn" – this means that your body continues burning calories for 46 hours after your workout.

Interval training sure beats normal cardiovascular training. Also, normal cardiovascular exercise usually takes longer as the objective is endurance. Contrast this with interval training which only requires 30 minutes or less and which delivers significant results in just a few weeks.

While you will be choosing your specific exercises for the strength and resistance training and interval training, I will be recommending an exercise schedule and giving you tips for your best application of the exercises.

Below would be the best weekly schedule for your workout:

Day 1: Strength and resistance exercises

Day 2: Interval training exercises

Day 3: Strength and resistance exercises

Day 4: Interval training exercises

Day 5: Strength and resistance exercises

Day 6: Interval training exercises

Day 7: Rest

As you can see, strength exercises and interval training are done on alternate days. This is to facilitate recovery of the muscles you use. Do not ever do your strength exercise workout right after your interval training workout – this will slow down the process of muscle building.

One day without exercise during the week is also crucial for your body to make a full recovery.

Again, I would like to emphasize that you should never push your body to fatigue. Doing so would trigger a stress response in your body, which may have serious effects on your metabolism. (The link between stress and metabolism will be discussed in a later section). Also, make sure that you breathe normally throughout the exercises so that your body is not stressed.

Always perform warm-up exercises before your routine and cool-down exercises after. For a warm-up, a cardio of moderate intensity and arm circling would be a good example. For a cool-down, a total body stretch will relax your muscles. Breathing exercises will also help in relaxing.

You can apply variety to your exercise routines to work different muscles and for your own enjoyment, especially if you get bored with the same exercise routines.

A Few Notes on Exercise to Boost the Metabolism

Here are some more things to think about as you plan your exercise program to fire up your metabolism:

1. Age does not matter. Yes, whether you are 20 or 60, you can trust that the exercise program we discussed will work for you. For older people, your interval training may not be as intense at first, but after some time, you just might be surprised how far your body can go. Looking at strength and resistance training in particular: here's something for older people to consider: a scientific study conducted at Tufts university shows that age is not an obstacle to building muscle. In their study, 87- to 96-year-old women who underwent an 8-week strength training program tripled their strength and increased their muscle by ten percent.

2. Other exercise is good, but... I recommend you apply the exercise program discussed here. While it is true that any physical activity burns calories, it only has a one-time effect. The

exercises here, however, are guaranteed to have a long-term effect. Also, endurance training is good, but you will get more and faster results from interval training.

3. More exercise does not mean faster metabolism. Logically, more exercise means more calories burned. But as your goal here is a long-term increase in your metabolism, you should not be obsessed by how much you exercise but on the quality of your exercise. Again, this deserves repetition – do not push yourself beyond your limits as it will drive your body into a stress reaction. Stress has a serious effect on metabolism.

So now you know the best exercise program to fire up your metabolism. But don't stop reading just yet – exercise is only one part of your journey to a faster metabolism.

CHAPTER 5- YOUR LIFESTYLE AND ITS EFFECTS ON METABOLISM

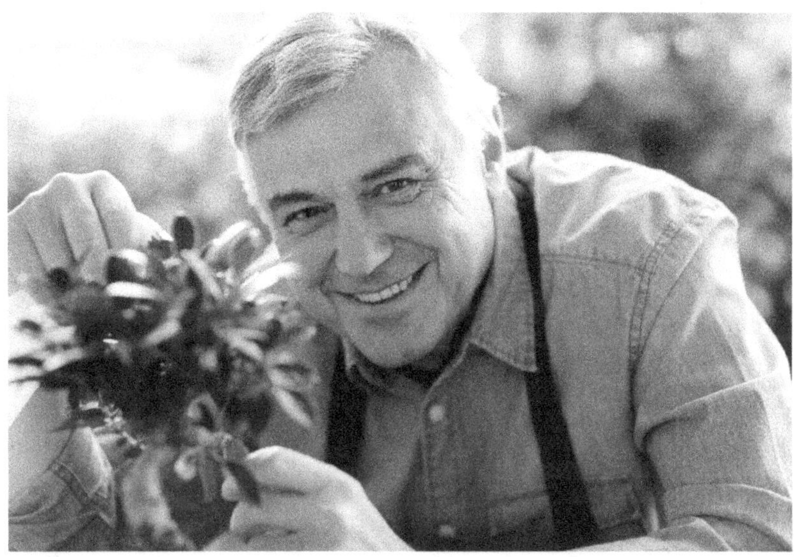

Balancing work, family, hobbies, and other commitments often means that our lifestyle isn't so much a choice, as it is a necessity, but we can do little things that help speed up our metabolism.

Follow Your Idols' Footsteps

Do you know people who carefully choose low-fat, low-calorie meal choices, are very disciplined when it comes to resisting the Chef's Special pecan pie for desert, yet order a glass or two of wine with their meal?

These people are undermining their efforts to boost their metabolism.

Studies show that drinking alcohol with meals actually encourages over eating, which means more calories that need to be burned away or transformed into fat.

Many people are simply unaware that many alcoholic drinks are laden with calories, almost as much as sugary soft drinks.

A bottle of beer or a cocktail is a few hundred calories. Wine is less, but still adds your calorie count. The tip here isn't to stop drinking alcohol altogether, but to be aware that it's adding to your calorie intake.

Ladies Become Fat-Burning Machines When They Bleed

Scientists have determined that the 2-week period prior to menstruation is a premium fat burning time. Australian studies have shown that women were able to burn off as much as 30% more fat in the 2 weeks preceding their period.

At this time, the female body's production of estrogen and progesterone are at their highest. Since these hormones tell the body to use fat as a source of energy, exercising during this time can really pay off. The body will be inclined to target fat cells for catabolism.

Calories are Your Friends

The word calorie has a bad rap. We constantly come across calorie reduced or low calorie foods.

The calories that come from cake are empty calories, which means there's no real nutritional value that your body can squeeze out and make use of. But in the bigger picture, it's unwise for your metabolism to become calorie-avoidant.

If you suddenly decrease the amount of calories that you eat, your body won't try to do more with less. It won't necessarily provoke catabolism and thus reduce weight and fat cells. Instead, your body will try to keep you alive by slowing down its metabolism. It will simply believe that something is wrong, maybe you're trapped somewhere without food, and it will just begin to become very stingy with energy.

So what's the end result? If your body needs 2000 calories a day to survive, and you suddenly give it only 1000, it won't begin to burn off 1000 calories worth of cells that you have lying around on your love handles.

Instead, your body will slow down its metabolism. It will really try and get as much energy out of those 1000 calories as it can, because it doesn't want to waste anything.

You'll feel more tired because your body is being very miserly with energy, and will devote its 1000-calorie ration to essential systems, like blood and oxygen supply.

Metabolically, you won't be burning off extra calories. In fact, you can actually gain weight by dramatically reducing your calorie intake.

The flipside of this is you should consume a daily caloric intake that is proportionate to your body size, type, and weight loss goals.

Once you determine the amount of calories that you need, you can provide that to your body via healthy, efficient calories. For example, if your body needs 1500 calories per day, and one slice of double-fudge chocolate cake delivers 500 of those, you can see that eating just one slice will take up a full 1/3 of your daily caloric needs, and that's not good.

On the other hand, you can see that drinking a tasty fruit smoothie made with yogurt and nuts can deliver half as many calories, but provide you with essential nutrients, vitamins, and other elements that your body needs to healthily do its work.

De-Stress When Needed

We now live in a fast-paced culture driven by urgency and deadlines. The more things you get done in less time, the better. Work, family and recreation have become a balancing act. Tension, worry, anxiety and fear are all too common. Emotional problems like failure in marriages, deaths of loved ones, or simply troubled relationships are accompanied with pressures from work.

Stress, especially prolonged exposure to stress, can seriously affect your metabolism, as well as your overall health and well-being.

How Does Stress Affect Your Metabolic Health?

There is a hormone in our body called cortisol, which aids in certain body functions. It aids regulation of blood pressure, release of insulin for blood sugar stability, increase of immunity, and proper metabolism of glucose. Small increases of cortisol can be beneficial, resulting in a quick, healthy jolt of energy and immunity, heightened memory, and a higher pain threshold. However, when too much cortisol is released or if it is released too often, it results in the following:

• Blood sugar imbalances

• Higher blood pressure

• Decreased immunity

• Lower cognitive performance

• Decrease in bone density

• Decrease in muscle tissue

Cortisol particularly stimulates amino acid release from your muscles to be converted to glucose that will serve as an energy source for your body to cope with stress. Yes, your hard-earned muscles are at the mercy of cortisol if you don't control its levels in your body.

The release of cortisol is mainly triggered by stress, whether physical or emotional in nature. Remember what we talked about for your exercise routine? Do not overtax yourself as it triggers the body's stress response.

Stress is also harmful to the body as it leads to the production of more acid than the body needs. Our bodies usually have an 80 percent alkaline and 20 percent acid balance. More acid in the body will upset that balance. Too much acid decreases your immunity and makes you more vulnerable to illness. Too much acid also affects body functions, including metabolism.

You can effectively cope with stress and keep your cortisol levels healthy and stable, though. When your body goes into the stress response, it is important that you help it go into the relaxation response.

How to De-stress

There are many ways to de-stress, as there are many causes of stress. Pick the ones to your liking.

Boost Your Metabolism in 45 Minutes
To re-charge, try the following:

1. Aromatherapy – This is particularly effective to let your stress during the day dissipate. Lavender and mint essential oils have excellent relaxing properties. A few drops mixed with water on your oil burner will suffice. You can also combine aromatherapy with meditation. As the aroma envelops you, feel it slowly sucking in your tiredness and worries. As the aroma leaves later on, imagine that your tiredness and worries are also going away with it. You can also briefly relax with aromatherapy during work. Put a few drops on a piece of tissue paper and inhale. Close your eyes while doing this.

2. Massage – This is also aptly called touch therapy. A massage is also beneficial as it loosens the muscles and joints that may have tensed up due to continuous stress. Back muscles are particularly susceptible to this. You can also combine massage with aromatherapy – you can ask the masseur or masseuse to use essential oils for your massage. Peppermint is particularly excellent. Aside from its aroma, it has a cooling effect on the body when used as massage oil.

3. Music therapy – Put some gentle, relaxing music on your player, sit or lie in a comfortable position, close your eyes, and let the music wash over you. Imagine it washing away your worries, fears, and anxieties. A good alternative to soothing music is the sounds of nature, like ocean waves. Recordings of nature sounds are available in music stores. If you find you enjoy relaxing on the beach, then bring the beach home with you through a recording of ocean waves.

4. Imagery – Imagine that you are a kite slowly rising and floating through the air. You float in the bright blue sky in perfect balance and harmony with the wind. After some time, feel yourself slowly

gliding downwards and then softly touching the ground. The above imagery is particularly helpful not only for relaxing but for simulating a good response to stress – notice that the motion of the kite is in harmony with the wind, when the same wind can also make the kite spin out of control.

Another imagery technique is to imagine a beautiful scene from nature like a mountaintop, a secluded island, or a tropical rainforest. Imagine yourself, from a first-person perspective, walking through the place and taking in all the beauty.

You can vary the place you visit every time you use this technique, or you can pick one and make it your sanctuary – the place you flee to during moments of stress.

For long-term use:

1. Think positive! – Thoughts greatly influence your health and well-being. Your thoughts can actually manifest into reality, as maintained by philosophers, contemporary speakers and even scientists. Therefore, bad thoughts can manifest negatively while positive thoughts manifest positively. So if you are going to think, you might as well think of pleasant things. If you have anxieties over something, like an upcoming presentation for work, imagine yourself – from the first-person perspective – giving an excellent, flawless presentation. Imagine the reactions of your audience. Feel the feelings as if you were there already. Images are more powerful than words, so apply the same principle to your thoughts.

2. Let go of negative feelings. Wallowing in negative feelings equals more acid in the body. No wonder tension and fear lead to heartburn or indigestion while chronic worry and/or resentment makes you more susceptible to high blood pressure.

However, do not suppress your feelings, even though some may appear irrational to you. Doing so also leads to higher acid levels in your body. Feel the feeling, express it through healthy catharsis in a safe environment if you feel the need to (e.g. screaming into a pillow) – and let it go. Yes, the key here is to let go. Do not dwell on negative feelings.

3. Meditate daily – Make meditation a habit. In the long term, meditation brings you peace of mind and makes you more able to cope with stress. It need not be a complex meditation – stillness and emptiness of mind is the key. Sit in a comfortable position and breathe slowly, deeply. Focus on each part of your body and feel it release its tension. After you feel sufficiently relaxed, you can silently repeat a simple word with no particular emotional attachment for you – for example, you can say "tree." Or, you can actually say a letter, like a. Repeat this word or letter in your mind for about one minute. Then sit still and let thoughts come to your mind. Observe your thoughts as if you were apart from them, as though they were another person's thoughts. This is so that you do not dwell on any thought. Just objectively, naturally, allow any thought to enter your mind then leave. If you reach a state of emptiness, where you feel you are thinking about nothing, congratulations! It may take some time for you to reach this point, though.

4. Take up yoga. Not only is this an excellent stress-buster, it also directly fires up your metabolism. The endocrine system and the thyroid help regulate metabolism. Yoga has many positions which give a healthy twist and compression to your endocrine organs, thereby strengthening them for metabolism.

For relaxation from stress, though, a good yoga position is the corpse pose. As its name instructs, you should lie like a corpse.

Release all tension from your body. The corpse pose is actually a good ending to your yoga routine.

5. Plan ahead – If the cause of your stress is recurring, plan ahead. After you have identified the cause of your stress, ask yourself if there is any way you can avoid it. For example, one cause of your stress may be the morning rush-hour traffic. To be relaxed while you are on your way to work, you have to leave early. Then you remember you watch television every night, sometimes late into the night. To avoid stress in the morning, you conclude you can decrease your television time and go to sleep earlier the night before.

By the way, if your body is subjected to stress such as long working hours, you should modify your diet while still keeping the principles of the fast metabolism diet. You especially need Vitamin C, as this helps the body cope during stress. Load up on citrus fruits and strawberries. For vegetables, sweet red pepper is an excellent source of Vitamin C. Other than that, your diet remains the same – load up on complex carbohydrates, particularly fibrous ones and take in protein.

Why is Sleep Important?

Sleep is the time your body fully recovers from your workouts. This is also the time that your muscles grow – yes, they do not grow during your workout but while you are in bed. With little sleep, your muscles grow very little even if you put in much effort in your workouts.

Lack of sleep will also prevent your body from being in top form and will thus also affect your energy for workouts. You might find yourself getting tired easily even after a few sets or reps.

Also, scientific studies show that lack of sleep affects carbohydrate metabolism. Glucose is not metabolized as much, resulting in increased hunger and decreased overall metabolism.

It is important for you to get at least eight hours of sleep every night for the body to fully re-charge for the next day. Although people's circadian rhythms may differ, the normal circadian rhythm is 10 pm to 6 am. This is the best period for muscles to grow. So sleep early to increase your metabolism!

Some Important Reminders

For some, de-stressing may be the most difficult part of the program to boost metabolism. What if stress has become so much a part of your daily life that making serious changes in your lifestyle is difficult? You can take things slowly. The least you need to do, though, is to find some quiet time to yourself every day. It can be as little as ten minutes. Use those ten minutes to just relax and meditate.

Meditation goes a long way. Even ten minutes every day helps you cope better with stress. Studies show that people who meditate regularly are less stressed and are more able to meet life's demands. If there are times you cannot avoid staying up late, catch up on sleep on the weekend. Don't let your sleep "debt" accumulate. Sleep "debt" leads to poor cognitive function and poor health overall. Your body processes don't function as well as they should – and that includes metabolism. Take time to de-stress. It not only boosts your metabolism but also improves your health in general.

Chapter 6- Don't Eat Less, Just Eat Right

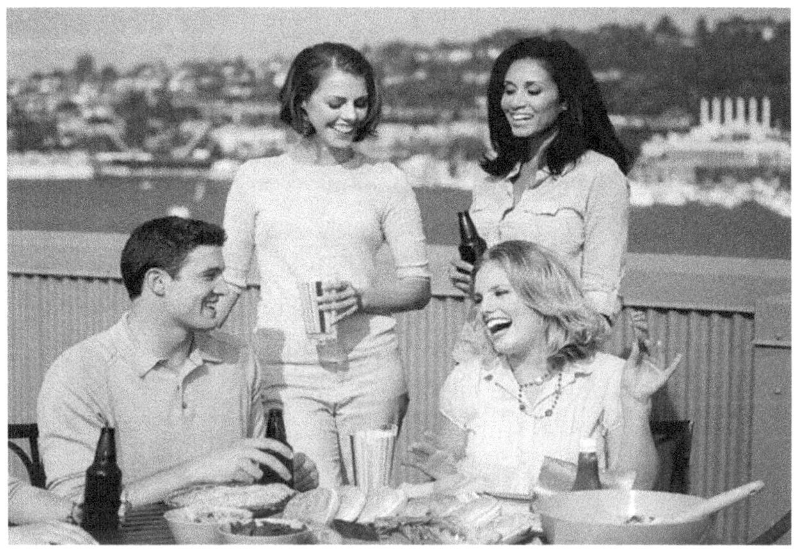

Food is your main fuel for energy – it gives your body the calories it processes to burn or to store energy. The right food, the right amount, and the right time in eating will give you the best results possible for your metabolism.

For all those who are trying to lose weight, you need to know that eating to boost metabolism is radically different from traditional weight loss diets. In traditional diets, calories are your enemy and you have to monitor your calorie intake, but the opposite is true for the fast metabolism diet. Calories are now your friends – the good calories, at least.

Remember when we talked about exercise? The more muscles you build, the more calories you burn. And after you've done interval training for a while, your body also burns more calories. So to keep up with the calorie burning, you actually have to eat more. You will understand this better later.

Nutrients to Love

Carbohydrates are one of the most essential nutrients for firing up your metabolism. They are the most basic fuel for the energy you consume for physical activities. If you exercise regularly, carbohydrates are necessary. But if you are building muscle, carbohydrates are crucial. As you progress in your muscle building and interval training, you need to increase your carbohydrate intake. As your body burns more energy, it will need more energy from carbohydrates. If the carbohydrates you consume are not enough, your body will turn to your muscle mass and get its energy there. Yes, your hard-worked muscles will be wasted if you do not consume enough carbohydrates.

More than 50 percent of your calorie requirements should come from carbohydrates.

There are two types of carbohydrates – simple and complex. Simple carbohydrates are easier to digest and absorb compared with complex carbohydrates. If we are to consider the thermic effect of food which also contributes to faster metabolism, complex carbohydrates are the way to go. And usually, complex carbohydrates are the healthy types of food while the simple carbohydrates are usually the processed foods loaded with preservatives and artificial sweeteners.

But simple carbohydrates should not be neglected entirely. Healthy sources of simple carbohydrates are honey, milk and fresh fruit juice.

Yes, carbohydrates are not all grains and root crops. We have fibrous carbohydrates as well – the vegetables. The fiber, though not absorbed by the digestive system, helps in the thermic effect.

Fiber also cleanses the body and thus ensures its smooth functioning, including the enzymes and hormones for metabolism.

Protein is another essential nutrient in the diet for faster metabolism. Protein is processed by the body into amino acids, the building block for cells – and consequently, muscles. And, like complex carbohydrates, protein also has a thermic effect as it takes a long time for the body to break it down.

Below are some healthy, excellent sources of protein:

1. Chicken – Go for the breast, as it has the highest amount of protein. Drumsticks are also good, though not so high in protein. Just remove the skin to get rid of saturated fat and cholesterol.

2. Fish – This is good protein without the bad, unlike red meat. Aside from having high protein content, it is also good for the heart, particularly cold-water fish like salmon and tuna.

3. Eggs – Very rich in protein and affordable too. Eggs contain all the essential amino acids for growth. Contrary to what some may think, the high protein content comes mostly from the egg white and not the egg yolk.

4. Milk – This is a must for anyone who wants to build muscle. It is no wonder that babies and toddlers are given milk for growth. So learn from your childhood and drink milk.

5. Whey – Though not a natural whole food, whey is very high in protein and is also healthy. It is a staple among body builders. Whey is sold as protein powder.

Fats are also essential for fast metabolism. Now, this may raise a few eyebrows, especially among those who have tried conventional weight loss diets. This is where the fast metabolism diet, again, sets itself apart. While too much fat – especially unhealthy fat – is bad, a small amount of healthy fats helps hormones responsible for metabolism to continue performing well. Diets low in fat lead to poor hormone production, and thus, slower metabolism.

When adding fats to your diet remember to keep them in their proper place: at the top of the food pyramid. Healthy sources of fat are olive oil, avocados, sunflower seeds, and nuts.

As with fats, calcium helps release hormones that boost metabolism. Milk, of course, is the best source of calcium. Yogurt is also high in calcium and has other health benefits as well.

"Nutrients" to Avoid

Avoid empty calories like the plague. These come from refined, highly processed foods – usually the simple carbohydrates that are not natural whole foods. Why empty calories? They fill you up but give little or no nutrients. What's more, these foods usually contain a lot of sugar – and too much sugar seriously affects the metabolism.

Too much caffeine is also not good for your metabolism. It triggers a stress response. So go easy on the coffee.

Other Recommended Foods

1. Spices – Cayenne pepper and red hot pepper, in particular, contain capsaicin which is said to raise metabolism up to 25 percent for three hours.

2. Green Tea – It's not all about antioxidants. Taken regularly, green tea can increase the thermic effect of food. Research data gathered by the University of Geneva shows that green tea speeds up fat oxidation in addition to boosting metabolism. Green tea also has less caffeine than coffee, whose caffeine level may greatly affect metabolism. For those who do not like the bitter taste, green tea extract is available in capsule form.

3. Soy – A study conducted by the University of Illinois shows that ingesting soy protein increases metabolism. The soy protein was injected, though, and not fed to the subjects. While the study is not 100 percent conclusive, taking soy, with its healthy protein and immunity-building properties, will not hurt.

Water is Your Metabolism's Fuel

The old advice holds true for overall health as well as metabolism – drink at least eight glasses of water a day.

Dehydration affects metabolism through a drop in body temperature. This drop triggers your body to store fat to help increase or maintain your body temperature.

Also, as you will be doing more exercises, you need water to keep your energy levels. If you sweat a lot, you should drink more water – even more than the eight glasses.

Water cleanses the body of toxins and thus enables body processes to proceed smoothly, including metabolism.

Eating and Timing

Even though you are consuming the right foods, your results will be compromised if your timing is not perfect. Follow the advice below and you will get the best results.

1. Eat several meals a day, every two and a half hours to three hours. To really maximize the thermic effect of food, you need to eat more than the usual three meals. Eating every three hours will allow the thermic effect to last you throughout the day, as it takes between two and a half to three hours to digest food while protein broken down to amino acids stays for three hours in the bloodstream. For the exact number of meals, the magic number for men is six while it is five for women. Men require 600-900 more calories every day than women.

   Do not go over your optimal number of meals, especially through late night snacking. When you are asleep, your body has a difficult time digesting. Also, the calories from your last meal are stored as fat. Keeping the last meal light and easier to digest compared with the earlier meals is recommended.

2. Always eat breakfast. Your body has been in starvation mode during your sleep time. To get your metabolism up and running again, start the day right with a healthy, hearty breakfast. The later you eat your first meal for the day, the later your metabolism starts.

3. Do not skip meals. Under no circumstances should you skip meals, especially the three basic meals. If you have a busy schedule and have a hard time snacking, keep "emergency" foods within your reach, like whole wheat crackers and bananas. During particularly hectic days, just a few crackers or one banana

would suffice as a snack to keep your metabolism running. A fresh fruit shake or a protein shake would also be enough.

4. Take one snack or meal after your workout. A meal or snack with protein and carbohydrates taken within one hour after your workout for the day helps in the recovery of your muscles and the building of new ones.

5. Do not eat less than two and a half hours before bedtime. Though metabolism still happens while sleeping, digestion will be difficult and your calories will most likely be stored as fat in your body.

Sample Meal Plans

Below are two sample meal plans for a day. The key in each meal, particularly the main ones, is to combine protein and carbohydrates. Portions depend on your personal daily calorie requirements. Remember, though, that carbohydrates should have the biggest share in your diet – and these include hefty servings of vegetables! – followed by protein. Calcium is also essential. Fats are the least priority. You can include green tea with your meals – six cups throughout the day is best.

MEAL PLAN 1

6 AM - Meal 1

- Oatmeal with banana slivers
- Poached egg

9 AM - Meal 2

- Protein Shake

1 PM - Meal 3

- Skinless chicken breast drizzled with olive oil
- Brown rice
- Steamed broccoli

4 PM - Meal 4

- Green beans
- Potatoes

7 PM - Meal 5

- Salmon fillet
- Sweet potato
- Cauliflower

MEAL PLAN 2

6 AM - Meal 1

- Egg white pancakes (only one or two yolks can be added)
- Choice of fruit/s – banana, blueberry and/or strawberries

9 AM - Meal 2

- Yogurt
- Choice of fruit

1 PM - Meal 3

- Vegetable curry
- Brown rice

4 PM - Meal 4

- Fruit salad with greens and
- grilled chicken

(Note: dressing should ideally be vinaigrette, with olive oil)

7 PM - Meal 5

- Chili (made of turkey, kidney beans and salsa)
- Steamed vegetables
- Milk can be taken as a last "meal."

These meal plans are here just to give you an idea. Create your own, but remember the principles. You can also change the times here, but remember not to eat too late at night.

A Few Reminders on Diet and the Metabolism

Below are just some caveats and some things to watch out for in eating and nutrition for faster metabolism:

1. Some foods can only take you so far. Spicy foods and green tea do have some effect in boosting metabolism, but only as an addition to a diet already rich in protein and carbohydrates. Relying on these alone for your diet for faster metabolism is not enough.

2. Some foods won't take you there at all. Grapefruit especially is popular among dieters as its high acidity is perceived to burn fats. However, there is no scientific proof for this.

3. No supplement will boost your metabolism. To those who are taking supplements to boost your metabolism, you may just be

wasting your money. Again, there is no scientifically proven link between supplements and faster metabolism.

4. Diet pills are a no-no. For those who want to lose weight, some diet pills may burn some fat and control your appetite. However, they do NOT boost metabolism. Also, the downside of diet pills is that once you get used to a certain dose, you need to take more to get the same effect as before. A few of those diet pills out there may indeed boost metabolism, but can have serious side effects. Read the box or container carefully. Better yet, consult your doctor. Looking at the adverse effects diet pills can have, wouldn't you prefer to boost your metabolism the natural way? You will look and feel better.

CHAPTER 7- BUSTING MYTHS ABOUT METABOLISM AND DIET

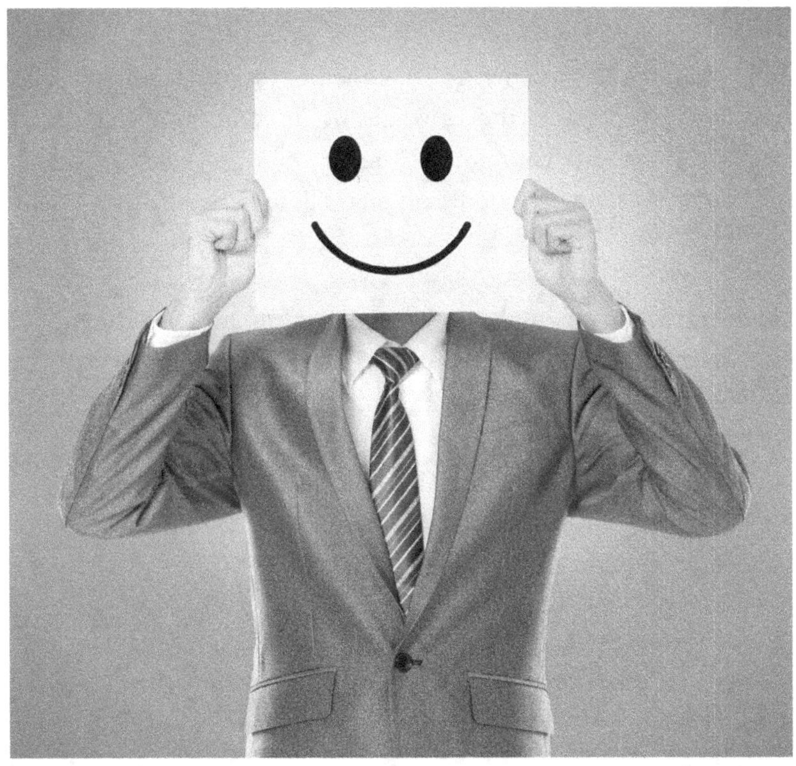

Myth #1: Diet Pills

The general consensus on diet pills are contained in two powerful words: BUYER BEWARE.

The problem here is that many makers of diet pills offer claims that simply aren't realistic; and if you read the fine-print of most of these advertisements, you'll see that they're really too good to be true. Little notes like the claims made in this advertisement are not typical should be enough of a wake-up call to realize that there's more to the story.

In some cases, diet pills can help boost metabolism temporarily. This, however, can be risky and generally shouldn't be done without a doctor's say-so. Unfortunately, people can become somewhat addicted to diet pills, and this can lead to disaster.

And before we go onto myth #2, remember that some diet pills are water loss pills. That is, they are diuretics that promote water loss, usually through excess urination. The jury on water-loss diet pills is somewhat less open-minded than diet pills in general: THEY DON'T WORK!

Seriously: water loss diet pills are built on the premise that you'll lose weight through water. And, yes, that's true: if you urinate 15 times a day, you're physically going to weigh less.

But this is not actual weight loss! This is merely unhealthy temporary weight loss, and it will come roaring back the minute that water stores are replenished through diet.

Or, even harder to comprehend, if a person taking these water pills fails to restore their body's fluid needs, they can actually suffer dehydration; which can, and has, led to coma and death.

Myth #2: Drop Caloric Intake

As we discussed earlier in this book (but it's so important that it deserves an encore here at the end), trying to lose weight by drastically cutting down calories doesn't work; in fact, it's unhealthy.

The thing to remember is that the body's ability to lose weight is not controlled by calories. Calories are the input. The real control mechanism is that famous concept that you've become very familiar with: metabolism.

Calories are merely units of energy. It's how your body deals with that energy that determines whether weight is gained or lost.

So with that being said, cutting down your caloric intake to, say, 1000 calories a day isn't necessarily going to help you lose weight; because it doesn't necessarily change your metabolism.

Indeed, as you know, if you slow down your caloric intake, your body – which is always trying to help you in the best way that it knows how – will slow down its metabolism.

Really, it makes sense: the body says that something has gone wrong; instead of the 2000 calories that it needs, it's only getting 1000. The body doesn't know why this is happening; it doesn't know that you want to lose weight.

It just senses that something is wrong; perhaps you're trapped in a cave or something, or stuck in a snowstorm. So the body, trying to help you, will slow down its metabolism; it will do its best to slow down the conversion rate, so that you have as much energy on hand as possible.

Now, if your body was able to read this book and you could say: look, please just do what you normally do, but do it with 1000 fewer calories a day for a while, then we might actually get somewhere.

But the body doesn't work that way. It won't help you lose weight if you dramatically cut down on calories.

It will slow down metabolism, and (here's the worst part), if and when you ever increase calories again, your body will have to deal with that via a slower metabolic engine. So you can actually gain weight if, after cutting down your calories for a period of time, you find that you consume extra calories (say while on vacation or something).

Myth #3: Low Intensity Workouts

It's fair to say that any exercise is better than no exercise. So if you lead a sedentary lifestyle, then even walking around your block for 10 minutes a day is going to something positive for your body and its metabolism.

True, that difference may be imperceptible to the naked eye (or it may not?), the bottom line is that exercise is good.

Yet with this being said, some people believe that they should perform low-intensity workouts even when they could be performing more high-intensity workouts.

That is, instead of jogging for 20 minutes with their heart at the top end of their aerobic zone, they opt for low-intensity jogs that barely break a sweat.

Low intensity workouts simply don't lead to a faster metabolism; they can't. Remember, as we discussed very early in this book, metabolism is a process.

And that process is really one of two types: taking energy and making cells (anabolism), or breaking cells down to make energy (catabolism).

If you don't achieve a high-intensity workout, your body can't tap achieve catabolism; it won't need to. And the only way your body is going to go and break down existing cells is if it needs to.

So keep this in mind as you exercise, either at home or at a gym. Low intensity workouts are better than nothing at all; and they may be necessary if you're recovering from injury, or just starting out on the exercise journey.

But once you reach a level of basic fitness, only high intensity (aerobic) workouts will make a difference in terms of your metabolism. High intensity workouts force your body to find energy to help you maintain that level of exercise; and it does so through catabolism.

Myth #4: Too Much Focus

Speeding up your metabolism and achieving your weight loss goals involved a certain degree of focus; after all, there's a lot of things competing for your attention (including that delicious Chef's Special pecan pie!), and you certainly need to be able to keep your eye on the goal in order to maintain your program. Yet sometimes too much focus can be a bad thing; and some dieters understand this all too well.

Remember: speeding up your metabolism is a holistic effort that includes exercise, lifestyle, and diet changes.

Focusing on only one of these at the expense of the others (either one or both) can be detrimental. In fact, in some cases, it can be counter-productive.

So the myth here is that you shouldn't go all out and focus on becoming an exercise guru, and then move onto lifestyle, and then to diet.

You have to integrate all 3 aspects into your life at the same time. True, based on your unique situation, you will likely emphasize one more than the others. That's fine and normal. But it's a myth – and a mistake – to ignore any one of these.

It takes all three to speed up your metabolism, and to get you to your weight loss goals for the long-term.

ABOUT THE AUTHOR

Charles Williamson is a fitness and wellness enthusiast who has built an empire manufacturing and selling gym equipment. Although the use of machines in attaining the perfect body for you is his source of livelihood, Charles remains to be very passionate in reminding everyone that the best machine to be fit is always free – and that is your own body.

Charles believes that with the right education, your efforts and hard work will pay off quicker and more effectively.

When not busy in his company, Charles would spend quiet afternoons with the love of his life – his wife, Marina.

www.ingramcontent.com/pod-product-compliance
Lightning Source LLC
Chambersburg PA
CBHW050702250726
48662CB00002B/798